# UNDERSTANDING PERIMENOAPUSE

## WOMAN IN PLENITUDE

### SUSAN MCDOWELL

THINKING SCHOOL

# UNDERSTANDING PERIMENOPAUSE

## Woman in plenitude

### - Susan McDowell -

Understanding perimenopause / Susan McDowell – 1st Edition

ISBN 9798321462560

# INDEX

# INTRODUCTION

Welcome to an extraordinary chapter in your story, a journey that takes us to explore perimenopause with curiosity, understanding and warmth. Perimenopause, that single transition stage in women's lives, is much more than a physiological process; it is a journey of self-discovery, acceptance, and empowerment.

Menopause is a natural and significant stage in a woman's life, marking the time when menstrual periods end, usually after a year without cycles. This transition, which is commonly experienced around age 50, follows the unique rhythm of each woman's body, with some experiencing these changes around age 45 and others continuing through their 50s.

The journey to menopause begins with perimenopause, a time of transformation that can begin as early as the late 1930s or as late as the early 1950s, extending over a period that usually lasts 2 to 8 years. During this time, it is possible to experience irregular periods and other symptoms, reflecting your body's natural fit.

Embracing menopause as a natural phase of aging is essential, and even if no treatment is needed unless symptoms are uncomfortable, learning about it can help. Understanding what is to come can provide peace of mind and support your well-being in this new life phase, allowing you to live it with health and serenity.

Imagine this period as a kaleidoscope of changes, where each twist reveals a new facet of your femininity. It is a time where emotions dance in harmony with hormonal cycles, where symptoms and body changes tell a unique personal story. We embarked on this journey not only to understand the biology behind perimenopause, but to embrace it as an opportunity to grow, learn and flourish.

In this warm and cozy corner, we will explore together every aspect of perimenopause. From clearly defining what it is to immersing ourselves in the nuances of its symptoms, we will unravel the secrets of this transitory phase. But beyond information, this is a space where experiences intertwine, where personal anecdotes connect us and where every woman, including you, is a unique protagonist in this fascinating story.

So, let us take curiosity and understanding by the hand, and embark on this journey together. Let us discover the beauty of perimenopause, embrace the authenticity it brings, and celebrate the strength that resides in every woman navigating this special chapter of life. Welcome to this space of discovery, understanding and growth!

Perimenopause marks a unique and often challenging phase in a woman's life, marking the transition to menopause. This period, which usually begins in quarantine, is characterized by significant hormonal changes that prepare the body for complete cessation of menstruation. During perimenopause, estrogen levels fluctuate, leading to a number of physical and emotional symptoms that can vary in intensity and duration.

This book aims to demystify perimenopause, providing clear and accessible information about its medical, emotional, and social aspects. As we explore this journey, we will address not only typical symptoms, such as hot flashes and changes in the menstrual cycle, but also emotional complexities and the influence on sexual health. Through a deeper understanding of perimenopause, we seek to empower women to face this period with knowledge, confidence, and the ability to make informed decisions about their health and well-being.

Perimenopause is more than just a prelude to menopause; it is a crucial phase that deserves our attention and understanding. This transition not only marks the gradual cessation of fertility, but also triggers a series of physical and emotional changes that can affect women's quality of life. By understanding and approaching perimenopause in an informed manner, we can demystify symptoms, reduce associated anxiety, and enable women to make more informed decisions about their health.

The importance of this transition period lies in the ability to empower women as they undergo significant changes in their bodies and minds. By providing clear knowledge and practical resources, this book aims to be a comprehensive guide that not only informs, but also encourages self-acceptance and health promotion during this unique stage of life. Perimenopause deserves to be understood not as an obstacle, but as an opportunity for personal growth and comprehensive care.

Understanding perimenopause is critical because it represents a once-in-a-lifetime transition phase for women, with significant implications for their physical and emotional well-being.

Understanding perimenopause empowers women by providing them with insights into the changes they will experience in their body and mind. This empowerment allows them to make informed decisions about their health and adopt strategies that improve their quality of life during this stage.

Lack of information can lead to anxiety and bewilderment in women who experience perimenopause. By providing a clear understanding of the symptoms and associated changes, it helps reduce stigma and negative perception of this natural process.

Perimenopause affects not only the physical body, but also mental health. Knowing about this phase enables women to recognize and address changes in mood, anxiety, and depression, thus promoting better mental health during this transition.

Understanding perimenopause facilitates effective communication between women and their health care practitioners. This enables a collaborative approach to address symptoms and develop personalized strategies that are tailored to individual needs.

Perimenopause serves as a reminder that aging is a natural process that all women will experience. By understanding and accepting this period, women can adopt a more positive attitude toward aging and focus on comprehensive health care.

Knowing about perimenopause can motivate women to adopt healthy lifestyle habits. From adequate nutrition to regular physical activity, these choices help not only to alleviate perimenopausal symptoms, but also to lay a solid foundation for long-term health.

Knowing perimenopause not only provides a sharp vision of this transition stage, but also empowers women to embrace it as a natural part of their life cycle, thus promoting healthy and satisfying aging.

# DIFFERENCES BETWEEN MENOPAUSE AND PERIMENOPAUSE

The transition to menopause is a unique chapter in a woman's life, marked by two key stages: perimenopause and menopause itself. Understanding the difference between the two is essential to navigate gracefully and knowledgeably through this natural journey.

For many women, menopause is lived with serenity, without significant problems, and can even bring a sense of relief by saying goodbye to painful menstrual periods and preoccupation with pregnancy; and also its transition to it - perimenopause. However, each experience is unique, and for some, this transition may be accompanied by challenges such as hot flashes, sleep disturbances, discomfort during intimacy, variations in mood, irritability, and feelings of sadness, or a mixture of these symptoms. In these cases, it may be comforting to seek the advice and guidance of a physician to explore lifestyle changes or treatments that may alleviate these symptoms, thus allowing you to live this stage with greater comfort and well-being.

Perimenopause, in the first place, is like the prelude to a symphony heralding change. This period, which can begin in the fourth decade of a woman's life, is a delicate compass in which the body gradually prepares to say goodbye to fertility. During perimenopause, hormone levels fluctuate, leading to an intricate dance of symptoms that may include changes in the menstrual cycle, sudden flushing, sleep disturbances, and mood variations. It is like a waltz in which the body and mind are intertwined in a unique choreography, announcing the next act.

Menopause, on the other hand, is the falling curtain, marking the official end of reproductive capacity. This moment comes when a woman has gone 12 consecutive months without menses. Although commonly associated with cessation of menstruation, menopause is much more than that. It is the closing of a chapter, but also the opening of a new stage in a woman's life, where wisdom and experience are intertwined in a unique symphony.

A useful analogy might be to imagine perimenopause as twilight, the gradual transition between daylight and darkness at night. Hormonal fluctuations paint a sky full of changing colors, heralding the arrival of a new phase. Menopause, on the other hand, is midnight, a quiet moment when the moon shines in its fullness, marking a new beginning.

It is essential to understand that perimenopause and menopause are not abrupt events, but processes that develop over time. Each woman experiences these stages in a unique way, and respect for this uniqueness is fundamental. As we immerse ourselves in these changes, embracing self-care, seeking support, and cultivating a deep connection with our own bodies become valuable allies in this journey. Menopause is not the end, but a new dawn, and perimenopause is the prolog that prepares us for the next exciting chapter in female life.

In this fascinating journey toward menopause, it is crucial to recognize that each woman is a unique narrator of her own story. Perimenopause, with its hormonal difficulties and the challenges it brings with it, is not only a physical journey but also an emotional one. Emotions can fluctuate as much as hormones, and it is completely normal to feel trapped in a tangle of changes. This period invites us not only to listen to our bodies, but also to tune in to our emotions, to accept them with compassion and to understand that they are as valid as the waves that caress the beach.

Menopause, on the other hand, invites us to embrace the power of transformation. It is a culmination, but also a new beginning. As we bid farewell to biological fertility, we welcome emotional fertility, a wealth of accumulated experiences that nourish the soul. It is time to cultivate patience with oneself, to discover new passions, and to reinvent the relationship with one's body. Instead of seeing it as the end of youth, we can regard it as a flourishing of authenticity.

Self-discovery becomes an invaluable compass during this journey. Menopause is not simply a destination; it is a continuous process of self-reflection and growth. Self-acceptance becomes a powerful tool, allowing us to embrace our scars and honor our victories. The realization that each stage of life has its own unique beauty helps us shed external expectations and embrace authenticity.

Perimenopause and menopause are interconnected chapters in the tale of a woman's life. The first, a symphony of gradual changes and the second, the melody of a new beginning. As we navigate these changes, let us remember that we are the authors of our own history, and that each chapter, with its challenges and triumphs, contributes to the masterpiece that is our life. With self-love, compassion and an open mind, we can transform this journey into a harmonious dance towards fullness and authenticity.

# UNDERSTANDING THE PERIMENOPAUSE

**P**erimenopause is a transitional period in a woman's life preceding menopause. Unlike menopause, which marks the end of menstrual periods, perimenopause is a gradual process that spans several years. It is important to understand that this is not a one-off event, but a phase in which the body experiences hormonal changes and adjusts to the transition to menopause.

During perimenopause, the ovaries begin to gradually reduce production of estrogen and progesterone, the key hormones in the menstrual cycle. This hormonal decline does not occur uniformly and can result in a variety of physical and emotional symptoms. By understanding perimenopause as a continuous process, women can better anticipate and manage the changes they experience, empowering themselves to embrace this phase of life with knowledge and confidence.

At the heart of perimenopause, we discover a transition period in a woman's life, where hormonal cycles dance, symptoms and body changes tell individual stories, and authenticity becomes the guide. It is more than a physiological phase; it is a journey of self-discovery, an opportunity to embrace evolution with acceptance and self-love.

During perimenopause, hormonal fluctuations can result in changes in the menstrual cycle, from shorter or longer periods to eventual cessation of menstruation. Symptoms such as hot flashes, night sweats, sleep disturbances, and changes in mood may manifest intermittently.

It is essential to understand that perimenopause should not be perceived as a problem, but as a natural phase in a woman's life cycle. This chapter will provide a solid basis for exploring in detail the various aspects of this transition period, enabling women to address this change with an informed and positive perspective towards their health and well-being.

Furthermore, it is essential to understand that perimenopause does not have a clearly defined starting and ending point, but represents a transition stage that can vary in duration from woman to woman. This process can usually begin in the 1940s, although the exact age may differ.

The duration of perimenopause is a highly variable and personalized aspect that defines the unique experience of each woman during this transition phase. Although there are general patterns, it is critical to understand that there is no rigid, uniform schedule for the duration of perimenopause.

Variability in the duration of perimenopause can be attributed to individual factors including genetics, general health, lifestyle, and reproductive history of each woman. Differences in genetic predisposition and hormonal health may influence the length of this period. Perimenopause usually begins in the 1940s, but the exact onset can vary significantly. Some women may experience changes in their menstrual cycles and related symptoms in the early years of quarantine, while others may notice these changes closer to menopause.

Generally speaking, the typical duration of perimenopause ranges from a few years to, in some cases, up to a decade before menopause. Complete transition to menopause is defined retrospectively after 12 consecutive months without menses.

Certain factors, such as overall health, stress level, physical activity, and nutrition, can influence how perimenopause is experienced and perceived. Women who maintain a healthy lifestyle may experience less intense symptoms and a shorter duration of perimenopause compared with those with less healthy habits.

Variability in the duration of perimenopause is closely related to how the ovaries gradually decrease estrogen and progesterone production. The individual hormone response determines the intensity and duration of symptoms as well as the time it takes to reach full menopause.

Because perimenopause is an individualized process, it is crucial that women be aware of their own changes and seek medical attention to manage symptoms. Regular monitoring and open communication with health professionals are essential to tailor specific management strategies to the needs of each woman.

## HORMONAL CHANGES IN PERIMENOPAUSE

In the smooth flow of hormonal changes during perimenopause, we recognize your body's unique symphony. Each fluctuation tells a story of transformation, and in this warm and understanding chapter, we will explore together the poetry of those changes, weaving understanding, and acceptance into each note.

Perimenopause is intrinsically linked to significant hormonal changes that profoundly impact a woman's body. These changes, focusing primarily on the sex hormones estrogen and progesterone, trigger a number of physiologic and symptomatic events. We will explore in detail how these hormonal fluctuations manifest themselves and their impact on perimenopause.

Estrogen, a key hormone in the menstrual cycle, fluctuates during perimenopause. Initially, there may be elevated levels of estrogen, which can lead to irregular menstrual cycles and symptoms such as tender sinuses. As perimenopause progresses, estrogen levels tend to decrease, contributing to menstrual changes and other associated symptoms.

Progesterone, another hormone essential for the menstrual cycle, also varies. During perimenopause, progesterone production may become irregular, affecting the regularity of the menstrual cycle. This hormonal irregularity may contribute to symptoms such as changes in menstrual flow and shorter or longer periods.

The combination of estrogen and progesterone fluctuations can trigger changes in the length, frequency, and regularity of the menstrual cycle. Many women experience irregular menstrual cycles during perimenopause, with periods that may become shorter, longer, or completely unpredictable.

Decreased estrogen levels may contribute to typical symptoms of perimenopause, such as hot flashes, night sweats, vaginal dryness, and skin and hair changes. These symptoms are linked to the influence of estrogen in different body systems. Decreased estrogen levels during perimenopause also affect bone health. Loss of bone density may increase the risk of osteoporosis. In addition, the influence of estrogen on muscle mass may contribute to changes in strength and body composition.

Hormonal changes not only have physical repercussions, but also affect emotional balance. Hormone fluctuation may contribute to mood changes, irritability, anxiety, and depression in some women during perimenopause.

Crucially, each woman's response to these hormonal changes is unique. Some may experience more intense symptoms, while others may have a smoother transition. Genetic, lifestyle and individual health factors influence the way these hormonal changes are experienced.

such as vaginal dryness and changes in the elasticity of vaginal tissue. These symptoms can affect sexual comfort and health, underscoring the importance of addressing intimate aspects during perimenopause.

In addition to changes in estrogen and progesterone, hormones produced by the adrenal glands, such as DHEA and cortisol, may also be abnormal during perimenopause. These changes can influence energy, stress, and the body's overall response to daily demands.

Hormonal changes in perimenopause affect not only the reproductive system. There are complex interconnections with other systems, such as the cardiovascular system, the nervous system, and the metabolic system. These relationships may have implications for general health and chronic disease management.

Detailed understanding of hormonal changes in perimenopause highlights the importance of a comprehensive approach to health care. Medical care that addresses not only hormonal symptoms but also emotional, gynecologic, and general aspects can significantly improve quality of life during this stage.

As we explore hormonal changes, treatment options, including hormone therapy and other non-hormonal options, will also be addressed. Understanding the benefits and risks of these interventions helps women make informed decisions about their health and well-being during perimenopause.

It is essential to note that hormonal changes are not static; they evolve over time. Understanding the dynamic nature of these changes allows women to adapt to separate phases of perimenopause and adjust management strategies as needed.

Open and ongoing dialog with health care practitioners is essential. Women should feel comfortable sharing their symptoms and concerns to receive personalized counseling and treatment options tailored to their specific situation.

## ONSET AND TRIGGERS OF PERIMENOPAUSE

At the beginning of perimenopause, where time becomes a mixture of unique experiences, we embrace the diversity of each beginning and discover the richness of the triggers. This is a cozy space to understand and accept, where each woman, in her uniqueness, begins her own journey of transformation. As we venture into the beginnings of perimenopause, we explore not only the passage of time, but also the triggers that mark this journey. From genetics to lifestyle, each individual element contributes to the unique symphony of this phase.

Here, in our corner of understanding and acceptance, we recognize that the onset of perimenopause is as diverse as the women who experience it. It is a time when the threads of biology, genetic history, and life choices converge, creating a personal and unique narrative for each woman.

Through this journey, we immerse ourselves in the richness of individual experiences and celebrate the variety of paths that lead to perimenopause. In this warm and understanding space, we honor the beginning of this chapter, recognizing that each woman carries with her a unique story, woven with the beautiful complexity of her own life.

Perimenopause usually begins in the fourth decade of life, with quarantine being the most common stage for many women to notice the first signs of this transition period. However, it is essential to understand that the precise onset can vary considerably among women.

Genetic factors play a crucial role in determining when a woman will begin perimenopause. Inheritance influences the age at which a woman's mother or sisters went through this process. Despite these familial patterns, individual variability is significant, and some women may begin perimenopause before or after their family members.

Hormone regulation is a key trigger of perimenopause. The gradual decline in the production of reproductive hormones, such as estrogen and progesterone, marks the beginning of this period. Changes in endocrine function, specifically in the ovaries, are crucial to understanding the onset of perimenopause.

Lifestyle also plays a crucial role in the onset of perimenopause. Factors such as nutrition, level of physical activity, and sleep habits can influence hormonal regularity and thus initiation of transition. Women who lead a healthy lifestyle may experience perimenopause more gradually and with less severe symptoms.

Exposure to environmental toxins, such as certain chemicals in food and everyday products, can also impair hormonal function and the onset of perimenopause. Studies suggest that the presence of certain endocrine disruptors in the environment may influence women's reproductive and hormonal health.

The reproductive history of a woman may impact the onset of perimenopause. Those who have had multiple pregnancies or have given birth to their children at a young age may experience the transition later compared to those with fewer reproductive experiences.

Chronic stress and psychologic factors may also play a role in the onset of perimenopause. Stress can affect hormonal regulation and contribute to menstrual irregularity and more intense symptoms during this transition phase.

Some chronic disorders and certain drugs can affect hormonal function and thus the beginning of perimenopause. Conditions such as diabetes or hypothyroidism can affect menstrual regularity, while certain drugs can have effects on hormonal function.

Because the onset of perimenopause can be influenced by multiple factors, it is critical that women undergo regular medical evaluations to monitor their reproductive and hormonal health. Open communication with health professionals allows early identification of perimenopause and implementation of appropriate management strategies.

## IMPORTANCE OF EARLY AWARENESS IN PERIMENOPAUSE

In the delicate fabric of perimenopause, the importance of early awareness reveals itself as a soft light guiding this journey. Recognizing the initial signs and understanding the subtleties of this transition period not only empowers, but also opens the door to more compassionate accompaniment. Early consciousness invites us to tune into our body and mind, to listen to the signals they send us. In this space of understanding and warmth, we embrace the truth that each woman is unique in her experience, and being aware early is like unfurling a personalized map to navigate this uncharted territory.

This early knowledge not only allows for practical preparation for physical and emotional changes that may arise, but also establishes the basis for a deeper connection with our own essence. Instead of being a mere bystander, we become co-creators of our history, recognizing that early awareness is a powerful tool to nurture wellbeing and vitality.

Here, in this space of understanding and acceptance, we celebrate the importance of being present in the first steps of perimenopause. It is an act of self-love, a commitment to self-discovery and an invitation to walk this path with grace and wisdom. In early consciousness, we find a valuable ally who accompanies us at every step, reminding us that this journey is ours, and that it deserves to be lived with compassion and self-love.

Early awareness of perimenopause enables women to identify and understand the first signs and symptoms that may arise. This includes changes in menstrual pattern, occasional hot flashes, sleep disturbances and mood swings. The ability to recognize these signs gives women an advantage in addressing challenges from the earliest stages.

Being aware of perimenopause, women have the opportunity to proactively address symptoms that may arise. Adopting self-care strategies, such as incorporating healthy sleep habits, practicing stress management techniques, and adopting a balanced diet, can help relieve symptoms and improve quality of life.

Early awareness also enables the search for emotional and psychologic support. Understanding the emotional changes that can accompany perimenopause gives women the opportunity to connect with mental health professionals, friends, or support groups. This facilitates emotion management and promotes mental health during this transition period.

Early awareness gives women time to educate themselves about perimenopause and its implications. With enough information, women can make informed choices about their health. This includes deciding on medical treatments, lifestyle options, and approaches to general well-being during perimenopause. Anticipating and understanding perimenopause early can help prevent the anxiety and stigma associated with this phase of life. Knowing that symptoms are part of a natural process, women can approach perimenopause with a more positive and empowered attitude, reducing negative emotional impact.

Early awareness empowers women to seek professional help when needed. If symptoms are significant or affect quality of life, consultation with health care practitioners provides treatment options tailored to individual needs, thereby improving perimenopause management. Early awareness involves not only identifying immediate symptoms but also preparing for long-term changes. Understanding that perimenopause is a transient phase leading to complete menopause enables women to take a long-term approach to their health care and well-being.

A.M., a 45-year-old marketing executive, discovered perimenopause by noticing changes in her menstrual cycle and experiencing symptoms such as hot flashes and sleep disturbances. Rather than being overwhelmed, he decided to approach the situation with determination and took a proactive approach. She adjusted her lifestyle, sought professional support, and shared her experience with friends, turning perimenopause into an opportunity to learn and inspire other women to face this stage with confidence and empowerment. Now, she is one of the people who leads and plays a facilitating role in working groups helping women like her.

Early awareness also means fostering a positive attitude toward the transition to perimenopause. By understanding that this phase of life is not an obstacle, but an opportunity for personal growth and adaptation, women can face perimenopause with a positive and proactive mindset.

Early awareness of perimenopause promotes continuing education about women's health. This includes being informed about medical progress, research, and resources available to address perimenopause. Keeping up-to-date facilitates informed decision-making and the implementation of more effective care strategies.

## PREGNANCIES AND PERIMENOPAUSE

Pregnancy during perimenopause is an interesting and complex topic because of the hormonal and reproductive changes that occur at this stage of a woman's life. Perimenopause is the period before menopause, marked by a transition in which ovarian function gradually declines, resulting in variations in menstrual cycles and hormone levels.

During perimenopause, although fertility decreases, it is still possible to become pregnant because ovulation continues to occur, although more irregularly.

As a woman approaches menopause, the number and quality of her eggs decrease, reducing the chances of conceiving. However, as long as menses are present, ovulation and thus pregnancy are possible.

Menstrual cycles may become irregular during perimenopause, which may make it difficult to monitor ovulation and thus conception. This irregularity can also lead to confusion about starting a pregnancy because missed periods can be mistakenly attributed to menopause.

Pregnancy in perimenopause may carry higher risks of complications such as miscarriage, gestational diabetes, pregnancy-induced hypertension, and chromosomal abnormalities in the infant. Therefore, close medical attention is recommended.

Women in perimenopause who become pregnant should consider their overall health, including factors such as chronic disease, lifestyle, and genetic risks, as these may impact both the ability to conceive and the health of the pregnancy.

Although pregnancy is possible during perimenopause, it comes with additional challenges and risks. Women considering conceiving at this stage should seek medical advice to fully understand their options and the care that should be considered.

# SYMPTOMS AND BODY CHANGES

In the symphony of perimenopause, the symptoms and body changes are notes that dance in harmony, each telling a unique story. In this space of understanding and warmth, we explore these changes with empathy, recognizing that each woman is a masterpiece in constant evolution.

In the chapters of symptoms and body changes of perimenopause, we immerse ourselves in an intimate journey where empathy and understanding intertwine. Every symptom, whether it is a fleeting hot flush or an alteration in the menstrual pattern, is a unique experience, and here, in our acceptance corner, we celebrate the richness and diversity of these changes.

From skin to weight, from bone health to vitality, we enter the very fabric of transforming femininity. These symptoms and body changes are like brushstrokes on the canvas of our lives, telling the story of perimenopause with a mixture of grace and resilience.

Instead of viewing these changes as mere challenges, we embrace them as intrinsic elements of life's wonderful symphony. Here, in this space where understanding meets warmth, we remember that every symptom is an invitation to explore, to care for and to nurture ourselves with love and compassion.

Thus, in this chapter of perimenopause, we immerse ourselves in the truth that every change, however small, is a testament to our inner strength and an opportunity to grow in acceptance of ourselves. With affection and understanding, we celebrate the poetry that resides in these symptoms and body changes, recognizing that, in every transformation, we are becoming more authentic and fuller versions of ourselves.

## HOT FLUSHES AND NIGHT SWEATS

Hot flashes and night sweats are two of the most distinctive and common symptoms of perimenopause. Flushing is characterized by a sudden sensation of intense heat that affects mainly the upper body, neck, and face. Night sweats, on the other hand, are similar episodes of excessive night sweats.

These symptoms are linked to hormonal fluctuations, especially a decrease in estrogen levels. Specific triggers may vary, but factors such as stress, certain foods or drinks, and changes in environmental temperature may exacerbate these episodes.

Hot flashes and night sweats can have a significant impact on women's quality of life during perimenopause. Interruption of sleep due to night sweats can cause fatigue and impair the ability to cope with daily demands.

The duration of these symptoms can vary widely from woman to woman. Some experience occasional episodes, while others can deal with them more persistently. Duration is usually most intense during perimenopause and may decrease after complete menopause.

There are several strategies for managing hot flashes and night sweats. From dietary changes to relaxation techniques and breathing exercises, each woman can find approaches that suit her specific needs. In some cases, medical options such as hormone therapy may be considered.

In addition to the physical impact, these symptoms can have emotional and psychological repercussions. Women may experience irritability, anxiety, or emotional problems related to sleep deprivation and physical discomfort associated with hot flashes and night sweats.

Many women find it useful to make lifestyle adjustments to reduce the frequency and intensity of these symptoms. This can include incorporating foods rich in phytoestrogens, managing stress through techniques such as meditation and regular physical activity.

## MENSTRUAL IRREGULARITIES

Menstrual irregularities are one of the most common signs of perimenopause. Women may experience changes in the length, frequency, and amount of menstrual flow. This may be manifested as shorter or longer cycles, lighter or heavier periods, and episodes of irregular bleeding.

Every menstrual irregularity in perimenopause is a note in the symphony of life, a unique expression of the transformation that is brewing. In this sanctuary of understanding and acceptance, we recognize that each woman carries her own melody, and menstrual irregularities are an integral part of this unique composition.

These changes, whether in the length, flow, or frequency of your menstrual cycle, are like flashes of light that illuminate the path to a new phase of womanhood. Here, in this space where empathy is intertwined with warmth, we celebrate the richness of these variations as testaments to your uniqueness.

Instead of perceiving these irregularities as deviations, we embrace them as authentic expressions of perimenopause. Every change in your menstrual cycle is an invitation to explore the connection with your own body, to understand its changing rhythms with love and patience.

These irregularities are related to the decrease of estrogen and progesterone levels, key hormones in the regulation of the menstrual cycle. As the ovaries begin to decrease in function in perimenopause, ovulation may become irregular, affecting the regularity of the cycle.

Perimenopause is a period when fertility begins to decline, and menstrual irregularities are an indicator of this transition. Women who want to conceive may find it more challenging because of irregular ovulation. It is crucial that those seeking to become pregnant seek specific medical guidance.

Along with menstrual irregularities, women may experience other related symptoms, such as more severe cramps, changes in texture and amount of discharge, and breast discomfort. These symptoms are varied and depend on the individual hormonal response of each woman.

Management of menstrual irregularities often involves adjustments in routine and lifestyle. Some women find it useful to keep track of their menstrual cycles to track patterns and anticipate changes. Adopting self-care practices, such as stress management and a balanced diet, can help mitigate symptoms.

For women who have not yet reached complete menopause and who want to avoid pregnancy, managing contraception can become more complex because of menstrual irregularities. Discussing contraceptive options with a health care practitioner is critical to finding the right one in each situation.

## SKIN, HAIR, AND NAIL CHANGES

In the soft embrace of perimenopause, changes in skin, hair and nails are touches of authenticity that reveal the history of your journey. Here, in our space of understanding and warmth, we celebrate these changes as visible manifestations of your inner strength and the unique beauty emanating from your being. Every change in your skin, every strand of hair, and every nail that grows in perimenopause is a tangible reminder of the wonderful transformation that you are experiencing. In this haven of understanding and acceptance, we honor these changes as external signals of internal evolution, where true beauty is woven from the inside out. The skin, which has witnessed every smile and tear, now reflects the story of your growth and wisdom. Hair, like a crown that adorns your being, carries with it the elegance of each lived chapter. And nails, small masterpieces that grow with patience, are witnesses to the strength that resides in your hands.

Here, in this corner where empathy meets warmth, we celebrate the authenticity of these changes in perimenopause. Beyond appearances, we recognize that every transformation is a precious aspect of your journey, an external expression of the strength, grace, and resilience that you carry within.

During perimenopause, many women experience a decrease in collagen and elastin production, which can lead to drier, less elastic skin. This can manifest as fine lines, wrinkles, and a general feeling of dry skin.

Hormonal changes may contribute to changes in skin pigmentation. Some women may notice dark spots or irregular skin tone, particularly on sun-exposed areas.

Although commonly associated with adolescence, some women experience an increase in sebum production during perimenopause, which can result in acne outbreaks. This change may be due to hormonal fluctuations and decreased estrogen production.

Hair loss and changes in hair texture are symptoms that some women experience during perimenopause. Decreased estrogen can affect hair health, making it thinner and prone to hair loss.

Nails may also be affected by hormonal changes. Some women experience their nails becoming weaker and brittle during perimenopause. This may be due to decreased production of keratin, the key protein in the nail structure.

Adopting a proper skin and hair care routine becomes essential. This may include the use of moisturizers to counteract dryness, sunscreens to prevent sun damage, and hair products designed to strengthen and protect hair.

## WEIGHT GAIN AND REDISTRIBUTION OF BODY FAT

Weight gain is common during perimenopause and is linked to hormonal changes, especially decreased estrogen levels. This weight gain is often located in the abdominal area, contributing to the redistribution of body fat.

Decreased estrogen can affect metabolism and the way the body stores fat. Lack of estrogen can lead to an increased propensity to store fat in the abdominal region, which contributes to weight gain in this area.

Perimenopause can also be accompanied by changes in metabolism, which means the body can burn calories less efficiently. This can make it harder to maintain weight or lose weight, even with previously effective dietary and exercise habits.

In addition to total weight gain, fat redistribution affects body composition. Muscle loss may occur, especially if resistance exercise is not routinely incorporated, contributing to a decrease in basal metabolism.

Hormonal and emotional changes during perimenopause can influence eating habits. Some women may experience more intense cravings or changes in food preferences, which may contribute to weight gain.

## IMPACT ON BONE AND MUSCLE HEALTH

During perimenopause, decreased estrogen levels may have a negative impact on bone density. Bone loss, especially in areas such as the spine, hips, and wrists, may increase the risk of osteoporosis and fractures.

Estrogen plays a crucial role in bone health by aiding in the absorption of calcium. Reducing estrogen levels during perimenopause can lead to decreased bone mineral density and an increased risk of bone health-related problems. In addition to bone health, hormonal changes can also affect muscle mass. Loss of estrogen may contribute to loss of muscle mass and strength, which may have implications for function and mobility.

The combination of muscle wasting and decreased bone density increases the risk of sarcopenia, a condition characterized by loss of muscle mass and strength. Sarcopenia can affect quality of life and functional ability. Resistance exercise becomes essential to counteract muscle loss and maintain bone health. Combining weight-bearing exercises or resistance training helps strengthen muscles and stimulate bone density. Diet plays a crucial role in bone health.

Adequate intake of calcium and vitamin D is essential to strengthen bones. Dairy, fatty fish, leafy greens, and supplements, if needed, can contribute to bone health. In some cases, especially if dietary intake is inadequate, calcium and vitamin D supplements may be recommended. However, it is important to seek medical guidance before beginning any supplement regimen.

Women in perimenopause should consider regular bone density examinations, such as bone densitometry, to assess bone health and take preventive measures if needed. Because loss of bone density increases the risk of fractures, especially in postmenopausal women, strategies to prevent falls and injuries are essential. This may include home safety measures and exercise programs that improve balance and coordination.

For some women, hormone therapy may be an option to address hormonal changes and protect bone health. However, the individual risks and benefits should be considered. Alternatives and personalized approaches should be discussed with health care practitioners.

In addition to resistance exercise, it is important to address muscle health holistically. This includes attention to nutrition, proper sleep, and stress management, as these factors can also affect muscle health.

# EMOTIONAL AND PSYCHOLOGICAL ASPECTS

In the intricate tapestry of perimenopause, the emotional and psychological aspects are threads woven with the most delicate emotions and thoughts. This chapter invites us to explore the inner landscape, where mood swings, anxiety and other emotional experiences intertwine with the depth of our essence.

We embrace every emotional high and low as an authentic expression of the human experience. We recognize that, in this phase, emotions can dance to a new melody, and each note is part of a unique symphony that is part of you.

Anxiety and a change in mood are not simply challenges, but opportunities to immerse yourself in a deeper understanding of oneself. In this space where empathy meets warmth, we celebrate the courage to face these emotional and psychological aspects, remembering that each woman is a hero in her own journey.

The importance of emotional self-exploration is magnified in this chapter. By recognizing and validating our emotions, we build a bridge to acceptance and self-reflection. Here, in this sanctuary where understanding flourishes, we encourage every woman to be her own ally, to listen kindly and to navigate the emotional tides with compassion.

In perimenopause, where the emotional waters may deepen, we remember that sharing our experiences is an act of connection and strength. Whether it is through conversations with loved ones, support groups, or seeking professional help, every step toward emotional openness is a step toward healing.

Thus, in this chapter that addresses the emotional and psychological aspects, we invite each woman to recognize the richness of her inner world, to embrace the complexity of her emotions and to find in this process an opportunity to flourish in authenticity and fullness. With understanding and warmth, we celebrate each emotional beat as a fundamental part of the evolving poetry that is perimenopause.

## CHANGES IN MOOD

During perimenopause, many women experience changes in mood due to hormonal fluctuations. These changes may include episodes of sadness, irritability, anxiety and, in some cases, depression. Hormones, especially estrogen and progesterone, play a key role in regulating mood. During perimenopause, decreasing these levels can affect brain chemistry, influencing how emotions are processed and managed.

Some women may experience more intense symptoms of depression or anxiety during perimenopause. These may include changes in appetite, sleep problems, lack of energy and a general feeling of hopelessness.

Physical changes associated with perimenopause, such as weight gain and changes in skin, hair, and nails, may have an impact on body image perception. This may contribute to the development of depressive symptoms and decreased self-esteem.

External factors, such as stress related to work, family, or personal responsibilities, may amplify emotional changes during perimenopause. It is important to recognize and address these additional factors to effectively manage emotional health. Women who have a history of mood disorders, such as depression or anxiety, may be more likely to experience more severe symptoms during perimenopause. Comprehensive mental health care is crucial in these cases.

Open, honest communication about emotional changes with friends, family, and health care practitioners is essential. Sharing these feelings can provide emotional support and contribute to a deeper understanding of the experience of perimenopause.

Practicing mindfulness and relaxation techniques, such as meditation and deep breathing, can help reduce stress and improve emotional well-being. These practices help cultivate mindfulness and manage emotions in a more balanced way.

Regular physical activity not only benefits physical health, but also has a positive impact on mental health. Exercise releases endorphins, neurotransmitters that act as natural painkillers and wellness generators. Incorporating activities such as walking, swimming, or yoga can be especially helpful.

A balanced and healthy diet plays a vital role in emotional well-being. Foods rich in omega-3, antioxidants and essential nutrients can have positive effects on brain function and emotional stability. Reducing consumption of caffeine and refined sugars can also contribute to a more balanced mood.

Keeping an emotional diary can help women identify patterns in their mood and better understand situations that trigger specific emotions. Regular monitoring of mood facilitates effective communication with health care practitioners and helps them make informed treatment decisions.

## STRESS, ANXIETY AND DEPRESSION

Stress can be intensified during perimenopause because of a combination of hormonal factors, physical and emotional changes, and daily responsibilities. Women may experience stress related to symptom management, work-life balance, and concerns about aging. Anxiety may increase during perimenopause because women may face concerns about health, body image, aging, and changes in family and work relationships.

Uncertainty about the future and adapting to new roles can be significant challenges.

Hormonal changes may contribute to depressive symptoms during perimenopause. Hormonal fluctuations affect brain chemistry, which can influence mood and perception of life. Depression may manifest as persistent sadness, lack of interest in previously enjoyed activities, and changes in sleep and appetite.

Physical symptoms of perimenopause, such as hot flashes, menstrual irregularities, and weight gain, may contribute to stress and anxiety. Perception of these changes may impair self-image and raise general health concerns.

Identifying specific triggers and triggers for stress, anxiety, or depression is critical. They may include life events, significant changes, interpersonal relationships, or work factors. Recognizing these triggers facilitates the implementation of specific coping strategies.

Developing effective coping strategies is essential. This may involve regularly practicing relaxation techniques, such as meditation or yoga, seeking social support, communicating openly with loved ones, and identifying activities that provide stress relief.

Psychologic therapy, such as cognitive-behavioral therapy (CBT), may be beneficial in addressing stress, anxiety, and depression. Therapy provides a safe space to explore thoughts and emotions, develop coping skills, and set realistic goals.

During perimenopause, it is crucial to establish clear boundaries and priorities. This means saying "no" when necessary, delegating responsibilities, and focusing on activities that promote health and well-being.

Self-pity is a key component in coping with stress and negative emotions. Learning to treat yourself with kindness and understanding, recognizing the shared humanity of experiences, can improve emotional resilience.

Taking a holistic approach to health involves addressing both physical and emotional aspects. Integrating healthy habits, such as physical activity, balanced nutrition, and self-care, contributes to overall well-being.

# SEXUAL HEALTH IN PERIMENOPAUSE

In perimenopause, the journey to sexual health is an intimate, delicate exploration. In this chapter of femininity, we immerse ourselves with understanding and warmth in the mystery of sexuality, recognizing that each woman navigates these waters with her own story, desires, and needs.

The hormonal changes that characterize perimenopause can influence the sexual sphere in many ways. In this sanctuary of empathy, we celebrate the diversity of experiences and understand that each change is an echo of internal transformation, where sexuality becomes an even more authentic expression of female identity.

Demystifying sexual health during perimenopause by inviting women to explore and communicate their needs with their partner and health care practitioners is essential. Here, where understanding meets warmth, we immerse ourselves in open conversations without judgment, recognizing that honest communication is the key to maintaining a healthy sex life.

Self-exploration and self-acceptance also become fundamental pillars in this chapter. In this space of support, we encourage every woman to discover and celebrate her own constantly changing body, to explore new forms of intimacy and to embrace the richness of sexuality throughout life.

Perimenopause reveals itself as an opportunity to reinvent and rediscover the connection with one's sexuality. With compassion and understanding, we honor the diversity of experiences and foster an approach that values sexual health as an integral part of overall well-being.

So in this chapter where sexuality is intertwined with perimenopause, we invite every woman to embrace her own sexual journey with acceptance and curiosity. We celebrate the authenticity of each experience and remember that, in this phase of life, sexuality is transformed into a beautiful and unique expression of femininity. With understanding and warmth, we explore together this sacred territory of sexual health in perimenopause.

## CHANGES IN SEXUAL RESPONSE

During perimenopause, many women experience significant changes in their sexual health because hormonal fluctuations and other factors can influence sexual response and intimate well-being. These changes, although natural, can present challenges and require deep understanding to maintain positive sexual health.

A key aspect of these changes is manifested in sexual response. Fluctuations in estrogen and progesterone levels may contribute to a decrease in vaginal lubrication, which can make sexual intercourse uncomfortable or painful. This symptom, known as vaginal dryness, can affect not only physical comfort, but also the quality of the intimate experience.

In addition, alterations in blood circulation to the genital region may influence the sexual response. Reduced blood flow can result in decreased sensation and excitability, which, in turn, can impair the ability to reach and maintain sexual arousal. Importantly, these changes are not limited only to the physical sphere, but can also have emotional repercussions and affect self-esteem and personal satisfaction.

Open and honest communication with the partner plays a key role in addressing these changes. Mutual understanding and willingness to adapt to new forms of intimacy can strengthen emotional connection. Also, exploring options such as lubricants or vaginal moisturizers, which can relieve dryness, and experimenting with techniques that promote intimacy and pleasure may be beneficial strategies.

It is crucial to keep in mind that each woman experiences these changes in a unique way, and what works for one will not necessarily apply to all. Patience with yourself and your partner is essential as you navigate through this phase of life. In addition, seeking professional advice, whether from a gynecologist or sex therapist, can provide personalized guidance and specific strategies to address individual concerns.

Perimenopause, far from being a stage to be feared in terms of sexual health, can be an opportunity to explore new forms of intimacy and emotional connection. With an in-depth understanding of physiological and emotional changes, as well as adaptive approaches and appropriate support, women can maintain positive and satisfying sexual health during this transition period in their lives.

In this context, it is essential to address not only the physical aspects of sexual health in perimenopause, but also the emotional and psychological aspects that can influence intimacy. Concerns about body image, self-esteem, and changes in the perception of sexuality may arise during this phase of life. Open and compassionate communication with oneself and with one's partner becomes a crucial component in addressing these challenges.

Perimenopause may also be associated with changes in sexual desire. While some women experience an increase in libido, others may face a decrease. These changes may be attributable to hormonal factors but also to emotional and lifestyle factors. Stress, fatigue, and everyday worries can affect sexual desire, and recognizing and addressing these aspects is critical.

Emotional intimacy is particularly important in this context. Cultivating emotional connection with the partner, focusing on emotional communication, and sharing expectations and desires can strengthen the intimate relationship. The joint search for solutions, experimentation with new ways of expressing sexuality and openness to adapt to changes are key elements for maintaining a healthy sexual life.

Sex therapy can be a valuable tool for couples who wish to specifically explore and address the challenges in their intimate lives. A specialist therapist can offer guidance, strategies, and a safe space to discuss concerns. Continuing education about sexuality in perimenopause, for both women and their partners, also plays a crucial role in understanding and accepting this stage of life.

It is critical to emphasize that sexual health is an integral aspect of overall well-being, and addressing changes in perimenopause not only contributes to women's quality of life, but also strengthens intimate relationships. By adopting a holistic approach that integrates physical, emotional, and relationship aspects, women can confidently go through perimenopause and maintain positive sexual health throughout their life journey.

## TIPS FOR MAINTAINING A HEALTHY SEX LIFE

Addressing changes in sexual health during perimenopause can be a challenging process, but there are strategies and practical advice that can help maintain a healthy and satisfying sex life during this transitional stage in a woman's life. The foundation for strong sexual health in perimenopause lies in open and honest communication with the partner. Expressing wishes, concerns, and expectations clearly encourages empathy and mutual understanding. The ability to adapt to changes together strengthens emotional connection and intimacy.

Perimenopause may be an opportunity for exploration and discovery in intimacy. Experimenting with new forms of pleasure, techniques and fantasies can add a positive dimension to sex life. The willingness to adapt and learn from each other contributes to an enriching intimate experience.

To counteract common vaginal dryness during perimenopause, lubricants and moisturizers may help. These products can improve comfort during sexual intercourse and reduce the chance of discomfort or pain. It is important to choose products that are compatible with individual physiology and preferences. Sexual health is intrinsically linked to general well-being. Maintaining healthy lifestyle habits, such as a balanced diet, regular exercise, and stress management, positively contributes to physical and emotional health, which is reflected in intimacy. Comprehensive self-care has a direct impact on sexual vitality.

Adapting to changes in sexual response takes time and requires patience. Self-imposed pressure can have a negative impact on sexual experience. Taking the time to explore, adapt, and communicate effectively is essential to building an evolving intimate relationship. Seeking help from a sex therapist may be beneficial for couples who face specific challenges in their intimate lives. Therapy provides a safe space to discuss problems, receive professional guidance, and learn specific techniques to improve sexual health.

Maintaining a healthy sex life in perimenopause often involves being flexible and creative. Experimenting with various times of day, positions, sex toys, or new ways of communicating can revitalize intimacy and keep the spark alive in the relationship. Emotional connection is a vital component of sexual health. Focusing on strengthening the emotional connection with the partner, through affectionate gestures, open communication, and the cultivation of nonsexual intimacy, contributes to an environment conducive to a healthy and satisfying sex life.

It is normal for sexual desire to vary during perimenopause. Adapting to these changes involves accepting that frequency and intensity can fluctuate and that this does not necessarily indicate a problem. Quality of intimacy and emotional connection may be more valuable indicators. Maintaining a healthy sex life during perimenopause involves a combination of mutual understanding, open communication, continuing education, and readiness to adapt. The key is to embrace change, experiment with new forms of intimacy, and cultivate a strong emotional connection that sustains a satisfying sex life over time.

## IMPORTANCE OF COMMUNICATING WITH A PARTNER

Perimenopause, marked by hormonal and physiologic changes, can have a significant impact on a woman's sexual health. In this context, the importance of open and effective communication with the partner becomes crucial. The transformation of sexual life during this transition period requires mutual understanding, patience, and the readiness to adapt to new needs and experiences.

First, it is critical to recognize that perimenopause can affect sexual response and intimacy in a variety of ways. Variability in sexual desire, vaginal dryness, and other symptoms may influence the intimate experience. Open communication allows the couple to understand these changes and address them together, fostering a supportive and understanding environment.

Honesty about one's needs and desires is essential in this process. Effective communication involves expressing openly and respectfully what is felt and needed in terms of intimacy. This includes a willingness to share concerns, desires, and expectations, creating a space where both partners can feel heard and understood.

Empathy plays a vital role in communication about sexual health in perimenopause. Both partners should strive to understand each other's experiences and emotions. The ability to put oneself in the place of the other facilitates emotional connection and promotes the construction of a solid intimacy based on acceptance and mutual support.

Adaptability to changes in sexual life is another key facet. Perimenopause may require adjustments in sexual practices, rhythms, and expectations. Open communication allows these adaptations to be discussed constructively, exploring together new forms of intimacy that meet the changing needs of both partners.

Shared education about perimenopause also strengthens communication. Understanding the normal aspects of this biological process and how it affects sexual health provides a basis for addressing the changes with knowledge and reduces the associated anxiety. This shared knowledge facilitates a collaborative approach to sexual health management.

The importance of communication during perimenopause goes beyond the physical aspects and encompasses the emotional sphere. Emotional intimacy is nurtured by open expression of feelings, emotional connection, and mutual support. Effective communication builds a bridge that allows to cross the challenges of perimenopause, strengthening the relationship and sexual health of the couple as a whole.

In a small town, Mary Diaz (M.D.) and Juan Pérez (J.P.) were a couple who had been sharing laughter, challenges, and unforgettable moments for years. They were both in the perimenopausal phase, a phase that, as they discovered, brought with it certain changes in their lives and in their relationship.

M., a vibrant and passionate woman for her work as an architect, began to notice changes in her menstrual cycle and some symptoms such as occasional hot flashes. At first, she was puzzled by these changes, but decided to research and educate herself about perimenopause. He realized the importance of communicating openly with his partner about what he was experiencing. J., a music teacher, was also going through his own series of emotional and physical changes. She realized that M. was going through a unique phase in her life and decided to be there for her in the best way possible. They decided to take a positive approach to perimenopause. J.P., always creative, surprised M. with special dinners and relaxed nights to counter daily stress. M., in turn, introduced mindfulness and yoga practices into his daily routines, which helped manage stress and improve his overall well-being. They also explored new forms of intimacy. They approached vaginal dryness in an open way and decided to try various products that would help them maintain a full and comfortable sex life. J. proved to be a supportive partner and together they addressed change; it is not one's thing.

Open and effective communication with the partner during perimenopause is essential to maintaining a healthy and satisfying sexual life. This communication creates a space where physical and emotional changes can be understood, accepted, and addressed in collaboration, thus promoting a solid emotional connection and sexual well-being throughout this phase of life.

# LIFESTYLE IN PERIMENOPAUSE

## ADEQUATE NUTRITION DURING PERIMENOPAUSE

The relationship between lifestyle and perimenopause is crucial for the health and well-being of women undergoing this transition. Within this framework, adequate nutrition emerges as a fundamental pillar to address physiological changes and maintain an optimal state of health during this period.

Hormonal fluctuations occur during perimenopause and may have direct impacts on metabolism, muscle mass, and body fat distribution. It is essential that women pay attention to their nutritional intake to counteract possible adverse effects and promote a healthy hormonal balance.

One of the key elements in nutrition during perimenopause is bone health care. Because women are more likely to lose bone mass during this period, adequate intake of calcium and vitamin D is essential. Dairy products, fish, nuts, and green leafy vegetables are rich sources of these nutrients, contributing to bone health and reducing the risk of osteoporosis.

Weight management also becomes an important consideration during perimenopause. Hormonal changes may influence fat distribution, increasing the propensity to gain weight, especially around the abdomen. Adopting a balanced diet, rich in fruits, vegetables, lean protein, and whole grains, along with regular physical activity, can help maintain a healthy weight and prevent associated problems, such as insulin resistance.

Also, perimenopause is often accompanied by symptoms such as hot flashes and night sweats. In this setting, some foods may exacerbate these symptoms, while others may help relieve them. Avoiding spicy foods, caffeine, and alcohol may help, whereas adding foods rich in phytoestrogens, such as soy, may help regulate hormonal imbalances and reduce the frequency of hot flashes.

Adequate hydration also plays a vital role during perimenopause. Vaginal dryness, a common symptom, can be mitigated by maintaining good hydration. Increasing water intake and eating foods that are high in water, such as fruits and vegetables, contribute to vaginal and general health.

Importantly, each woman is unique and may experience perimenopause differently. Consultation with a health care practitioner or nutritionist can help adapt nutritional guidelines to individual needs and ensure a balanced intake of essential nutrients.

Proper nutrition during perimenopause is a powerful tool to manage physical and hormonal changes associated with this stage. By taking a conscious approach to eating, women can improve their quality of life, maintain bone health, manage weight effectively, and minimize bothersome symptoms, thereby contributing to a smoother and healthier transition process.

## EXERCISE AND ITS INFLUENCE ON SYMPTOMS

The role of physical exercise during perimenopause emerges as a determining factor for the health and well-being of women in this transition stage. The benefits of exercise go beyond the simple physical condition; they positively influence the physical and emotional symptoms that can arise during this period, providing an integral tool to cope with perimenopause.

One of the highlights is the management of body weight. Perimenopause is often associated with changes in body composition and a greater propensity for weight gain. Regular exercise, including both endurance and cardiovascular training, can help maintain a healthy weight and counteract the muscle loss associated with aging.

In addition, physical exercise has a direct impact on hormonal balance. Releasing endorphins during physical activity can help improve mood and reduce the prevalence of emotional symptoms such as anxiety and depression, which often intensify during perimenopause. Physical activity can also help regulate sleep patterns, thus relieving the insomnia problems some women experience during this stage.

Strengthening bones is another crucial benefit. Perimenopause may increase the risk of bone density loss, increasing susceptibility to osteoporosis. Weight-bearing exercise, such as endurance training, is particularly effective in maintaining bone health, providing an essential component in preventing problems related to bone loss.

Vasomotor symptoms, such as hot flashes and night sweats, are common during perimenopause and can significantly affect quality of life. Surprisingly, regular exercise has been shown to be effective in reducing the frequency and intensity of these symptoms. Moderate physical activity, such as walking or doing yoga, may help control these symptoms and improve the overall sense of well-being.

It is essential to note that there is no single approach to the amount or type of exercise during perimenopause, as needs and preferences may vary among women. The key is to find activities that are enjoyable and sustainable in the long term. From dancing to swimming to weightlifting, the variety of options allows you to tailor exercise to individual preferences.

Physical exercise reveals itself as an integral component in the management of perimenopause. Not only does it influence physical fitness, but it also triggers a series of positive responses that directly impact the physical and emotional symptoms associated with this stage. By adopting a balanced and personalized approach to physical activity, women can not only maintain their physical health, but also improve their quality of life during perimenopause and beyond.

## STRESS MANAGEMENT AND RELAXATION TECHNIQUES

Stress management and the incorporation of relaxation techniques are crucial aspects in the approach to perimenopause, a stage in which women can face significant physical and emotional changes. The relationship between stress and symptoms of perimenopause, such as hot flashes and sleep disturbance, highlights the importance of implementing effective strategies to manage daily stresses.

Perimenopause, as a transitional phase in a woman's life, can raise concerns about aging, changes in body image, and adaptation to new circumstances. These worries, combined with hormonal fluctuations characteristic of this stage, may contribute to increased stress and anxiety. Stress, in turn, can exacerbate perimenopausal symptoms, creating a cycle that negatively affects quality of life.

Stress management involves taking a holistic approach that encompasses both physical and emotional dimensions. The regular practice of relaxation techniques, such as meditation, deep breathing, and yoga, has been shown to be effective in reducing stress and improving emotional well-being. These practices not only provide immediate relief, but also promote long-term resilience to daily stresses.

Meditation, in particular, has proven to be a powerful tool for reducing anxiety and improving mental clarity. Mindfulness, focusing on the present moment without judgment, can help women develop a greater awareness of their emotions and cultivate a more balanced response to stress. Integrating meditation into the daily routine, even for a few minutes a day, can make a significant difference in stress management.

Deep breathing is another accessible and effective technique. The practice of consciously breathing in slowly through the nose and out through the mouth can trigger the body's relaxation response, slow the heart rate, and calm the nervous system. This can be especially beneficial to counteract the physical symptoms of stress, such as hot flashes and muscle tension.

Yoga, with its combination of physical postures, conscious breathing, and meditative elements, offers an integral tool for stress management. Regular yoga practice can improve flexibility, strengthen the body, and reduce muscle tension, while encouraging the mind-body connection, helping women find balance during perimenopause.

In addition to specific relaxation techniques, it is essential to incorporate healthy habits into daily life. Regular exercise, a balanced diet, adequate sleep, and social connection contribute significantly to overall stress management and well-being during perimenopause.

Stress management and the adoption of relaxation techniques are essential elements to face perimenopause in a healthy and balanced way. These practices not only relieve the physical and emotional symptoms associated with this stage, but also promote a higher quality of life by providing effective tools to deal with daily stresses in a resilient and conscious way.

# PREVENTION AND HEALTHCARE

## IMPORTANCE OF REGULAR MEDICAL CARE

Regular medical care during perimenopause emerges as a fundamental pillar in the prevention and promotion of health at this crucial stage of women's lives. As they go through this transition, it is essential that women maintain a continuous relationship with health professionals to proactively address physical, emotional, and hormonal changes that may arise.

Regular medical examinations provide an opportunity to assess general health and address any specific concerns related to perimenopause. These tests may include blood pressure measurements, blood tests to evaluate hormone levels and metabolic health, and bone density assessments. These measures enable health care practitioners to identify potential health problems before they become more serious problems.

Assessment of hormone levels is particularly relevant during perimenopause. Because this phase is marked by significant hormonal fluctuations, understanding a woman's hormonal situation can help personalize medical care. This may include discussions about hormone treatment options or alternative approaches to address individual-specific symptoms.

Prevention of chronic disease is another crucial aspect of regular medical care during perimenopause. The risk of cardiovascular disease and osteoporosis may increase during this stage, and a preventive approach may make the difference. Discussing lifestyle changes, including diet and exercise, and the possible need for nutritional supplements with the doctor may be an integral part of the prevention strategy.

Mental health should also be part of comprehensive medical care. Perimenopause may be associated with mood changes, anxiety, and depression. These issues should be addressed sensitively and proactively during regular medical visits. Health care practitioners can offer guidance, recommendations for therapy, and, if needed, drugs to help manage the emotional aspects of this stage.

In addition, regular visits to the gynecologist are essential to assess reproductive health and discuss contraceptive options if needed. Questions about sexual health and vaginal function can also be addressed during these visits, providing a safe space to discuss topics that can sometimes be sensitive.

In conclusion, regular medical care during perimenopause is not only about addressing existing problems, but also about preventing possible complications and promoting comprehensive health. These consultations provide a platform for continuing education, individual risk assessment, and collaboration in health management during this transition phase. Maintaining a constant relationship with health care professionals is a fundamental step toward optimal well-being and quality of life during perimenopause and beyond.

## STRATEGIES TO PREVENT LONG-TERM HEALTH PROBLEMS

Preventing long-term health problems during perimenopause involves adopting holistic strategies that address both the physical and emotional aspects of health. This transition stage not only marks hormonal changes, but can also have long-term implications for cardiovascular, bone, and mental health. By implementing preventive strategies, women can strengthen their overall well-being and reduce the risk of health problems as they age.

One of the key strategies is to maintain a healthy lifestyle that includes a balanced diet and regular exercise. A diet rich in fruits, vegetables, whole grains, and lean protein provides the essential nutrients needed to maintain optimal health. In addition, regular physical activity not only contributes to maintaining a healthy weight, but also strengthens the cardiovascular system, improves bone density, and reduces the risk of chronic diseases.

Stress management is another crucial preventive strategy. Chronic stress can have negative impacts on physical and mental health, exacerbating perimenopausal symptoms and increasing the risk of cardiovascular disease. Incorporating relaxation techniques, such as meditation and deep breathing, can help reduce stress levels and promote emotional balance during this stage.

Bone health care is essential to prevent problems such as osteoporosis as women age. Adequate intake of calcium and vitamin D through diet and, if needed, supplementation, along with weight-bearing exercise, helps maintain bone density and reduce the risk of fractures in the future.

Prevention of cardiovascular disease should also be a priority. Perimenopause may increase the risk of cardiovascular disease, and adopting healthy habits such as regular physical activity, a diet low in saturated fat, and control of blood pressure and cholesterol are crucial preventive measures.

Mental health care should not be overlooked. Perimenopause may be associated with mood changes, anxiety, and depression. Seeking emotional support, whether through individual or group therapy, can be an effective preventive strategy to address emotional concerns and reduce the risk of long-term mental health problems.

Regular medical consultation, as mentioned above, plays a key role in the prevention of long-term health problems. Assessing individual risk factors, discussing preventive strategies, and maintaining a continuous dialog with health care practitioners can contribute significantly to the prevention and promotion of comprehensive health during perimenopause and beyond.

## PROMOTING MENTAL HEALTH DURING PERIMENOPAUSE

The promotion of mental health during perimenopause is an essential component for the overall well-being of women in this transition phase. This period, characterized by significant hormonal changes, can impact mental health, leading to symptoms such as mood changes, anxiety and, in some cases, depression. Implementing specific strategies to promote mental health becomes crucial to address these challenges and promote a positive emotional state.

A key strategy is to foster awareness and understanding of the emotional changes associated with perimenopause. Educating women about the relationship between hormonal fluctuations and emotional symptoms can help demystify these changes, normalizing individual experiences and reducing associated anxiety. Clear and accessible information about perimenopause can empower women to better understand and manage their emotions.

Promoting healthy lifestyle habits also plays a crucial role in mental health during perimenopause. A balanced diet, rich in essential nutrients, and regular physical activity not only benefit physical health, but also have positive impacts on mood and cognitive function. These habits can help stabilize energy levels, improve sleep quality, and reduce the risk of depressive symptoms.

Social connection and emotional support are critical factors for mental health during perimenopause. Establishing and maintaining strong social relationships can provide a valuable support system, allowing women to share their experiences, receive guidance and feel supported.

Participation in support groups, whether in person or online, can provide a safe space for expressing emotions and obtaining practical advice.

Self-care and stress management are essential elements in promoting mental health. Encouraging regular relaxation practices, such as meditation and deep breathing, can help reduce stress levels and improve the ability to cope with everyday challenges. Spending time on activities that provide pleasure and relaxation, such as reading, art, or music, can contribute significantly to emotional balance.

Seeking professional help is also an important strategy. Individual or group therapy can provide a space to explore emotional concerns more deeply and develop specific tools for coping with perimenopause. Mental health professionals can offer personalized guidance and effective strategies to address emotional symptoms.

The promotion of mental health during perimenopause involves a comprehensive approach that includes education, the adoption of healthy lifestyles, social connection, self-care and, when necessary, the search for professional help. By prioritizing mental health, women can improve their quality of life during this transition phase and cultivate a positive attitude toward emotional changes that may arise.

# CONCLUSION

In the fascinating journey of perimenopause, we immerse ourselves in a universe of changes, discoveries, and authenticity. This unique stage, marked by hormonal fluctuations, physical and emotional symptoms, invites us to explore the very essence of femininity in its evolution. But beyond the challenges, perimenopause gives us the opportunity to embrace authenticity, understand our changing body and mind, and cultivate deep self-care.

From the clear definition of perimenopause to the detailed understanding of its symptoms, triggers, and the importance of early awareness, we have unraveled the complexities of this transient phase. We explore the variable duration, the hormonal changes that shape the experience, and how to recognize the beginning of this individual journey.

As we delve into personal stories and made-up anecdotes, we have seen how women, like you and me, face this stage with courage and resilience. From lifestyle adjustments to strategies to manage specific symptoms, each woman weaves her unique narrative, contributing to the collective tapestry of perimenopause.

Deep detail about symptoms and body changes, as well as exploration of sexual health and emotional and psychological aspects, have distilled valuable information to navigate this journey with confidence and understanding. From hot flashes to mood swings, from bone health to sexuality, we have explored every corner of this phase with a warm, understandable approach.

Along the way, we have emphasized the importance of regular medical care, long-term problem prevention, and strategies for maintaining vibrant mental health. More than a biological process, perimenopause reveals itself as an opportunity for self-reflection, acceptance, and promotion of an integral well-being.

In this kaleidoscope of experiences, I invite you to embrace perimenopause as a unique transition into a new dimension of femininity. It is a chapter where authenticity becomes our guide, where self-care becomes a sacred priority and where we realize that, in every symptom and change, we are building our own narrative of strength and grace.

So, as you cross this bridge into the next phase, remember: you are resilient, you are unique, and you're weaving the most authentic story of your life. May your journey of perimenopause be full of self-knowledge, acceptance, and self-love!

# RESOURCES

Books:

Northrup, C. (2012). Cuerpo de mujer, sabiduría de mujer. Bantam.

Lee, J. R., & Hopkins, V. (2009). What Your Doctor May Not Tell You About Menopause: The Breakthrough Book on Natural Hormone Balance. Grand Central Publishing.

Ewing-Mulligan, M., & McCarthy, E. (2010). Menopause For Dummies. For Dummies.

Prior, J. C. (2006). Estrogen's Storm Season: Stories of Perimenopause. LifeTree Media.

Gittelman, M., & Prebil, L. A. (2006). The Wisdom of Menopause: Creating Physical and Emotional Health and Healing During the Change. Bantam.

Academic articles:

Santoro, N. (2016). Perimenopause: From Research to Practice. Journal of Women's Health, 25(4), 332–339. DOI: 10.1089/jwh.2016.6011

Randolph Jr, J. F., Sowers, M., Gold, E. B., Mohr, B. A., Luborsky, J., Santoro, N., ... & Korenman, S. G. (2003). Reproductive hormones in the early menopausal transition: relationship to ethnicity, body size, and menopausal status. The Journal of Clinical Endocrinology & Metabolism, 88(4), 1516-1522. DOI: 10.1210/jc.2002-021565

# ABOUT SUSAN MCDOWELL

In the dynamic world of health and wellness, Dr. Susan McDowell stands out as a visionary and a beacon of knowledge, profoundly dedicated to empowering individuals to reach their full potential. Her journey in medicine is not merely a career, but a lifelong pursuit of understanding and sharing the intricacies of human well-being.

Dr. McDowell's foundational expertise was forged at the prestigious University of Medicine and Health Sciences, where she earned her medical degree. This rigorous academic background laid the groundwork for a professional path characterized by a unique blend of hands-on clinical expertise and an unwavering commitment to research. For years, she has cultivated her own medical practice, earning not only the respect but also the deep admiration of her patients through her compassionate care.

Beyond the clinic, Susan McDowell has forged an innovative path as a prolific writer, extending her influence far beyond individual consultations. Her extensive writings are a testament to her profound medical knowledge, yet they offer something more: they distill her innate compassion and unwavering dedication to continuously improving the health and well-being of all who seek her guidance. Her publications resonate deeply, reflecting an integrative approach that has made meaningful contributions to the field. While the sources don't specify all her topics, the mention of "Going barefoot" alongside her medical background hints at the breadth and diverse nature of her explorations within health and wellness, reflecting her prolific output.

Through both her clinical practice and her impactful written works, Susan McDowell has firmly established herself as a highly respected figure in the expansive field of health and medicine, a testament to her holistic vision and relentless dedication. She truly embodies the spirit of a leading medical professional, constantly pushing the boundaries of knowledge for the betterment of others.

Beyond her impressive credentials and extensive knowledge, Dr. Susan McDowell's approach to healthcare is deeply rooted in her profound empathy and a genuinely warm, welcoming demeanor. Her clinical practice is more than just a place for medical consultation; it is a space where her deep passion for helping people reach their full potential truly shines through. This innate drive translates into an environment where patients feel not just treated, but genuinely understood and cared for.

Dr. McDowell's personal philosophy distills her compassion and unwavering commitment to the continuous improvement of the health and well-being of those who seek her guidance. It is this patient-centered approach, marked by a welcoming spirit and an admirable dedication, that has earned her not just the respect, but the deep admiration of her patients over many years in her own practice. While the sources primarily highlight her interactions with patients and those who seek her guidance, her demonstrated compassion and dedication suggest an intrinsically warm and supportive professional persona.

# OTHER BOOKS BY THE AUTHOR

"Andropause Exposed: The Hidden Male Menopause, Low Testosterone, and the Secret to Reclaiming Energy, Strength, and Confidence"

The groundbreaking book, "Andropause Exposed: The Hidden Male Menopause, Low Testosterone, and the Secret to Reclaiming Energy, Strength, and Confidence," offers a comprehensive, empathetic, and empowering guide to understanding, managing, and thriving through these changes.

"Parenting without fear: A Guide to Loving Your Children"

Are you tired of parenting approaches rooted in anxiety, control, or endless struggles? For generations, many parenting practices have been influenced by underlying fears: fear of children not learning, not behaving, or not succeeding. These methods, often relying on pressures, rewards, or anger, can be not only ineffective but also deeply detrimental to a child's intrinsic drive for self-development. In 'Parenting without Fear,' we invite you to embark on a revolutionary journey that challenges conventional wisdom and reconsiders the very foundation of how you guide your children.

"Going barefoot: natural running, walking and movement to respect your body"

In "Going Barefoot: Natural Running, Walking and Movement to Respect Your Body," Susan McDowell delves into the profound benefits of reconnecting with the earth through natural movement. This insightful book emphasizes the importance of barefoot activities in fostering alignment, strength, and overall well-being. Drawing from both scientific research and her rich clinical experience, Susan offers practical advice and exercises to help readers embrace a more natural way of moving.

"Understanding SIBO: The Enigma of Small Intestinal Bacterial Overgrowth".

This book, the result of Susan's clinical experience, offers a clear and practical perspective on Small Intestinal Bacterial Overgrowth Syndrome (SIBO). Through her work, Susan unravels the mysteries of this condition, providing readers with an essential guide to understanding, addressing, and overcoming SIBO.

"Understanding Perimenopause: A Woman in Plenitude"

Discover the beauty in every change, from hormonal aspects to symptoms and body changes. With personal stories and anecdotes that resonate, you will feel accompanied in this unique chapter of your life. It explores how sexual health, emotional and psychological aspects, and general well-being intertwine in a journey full of authenticity and self-acceptance.

"Complete Guide to Red Light Therapy: Optimal Health, Healthy Skin and Other Benefits of Red Light."

As an advocate of holistic approaches to health, Susan explores the diverse benefits of red-light therapy in this book. From improving skin health to optimizing overall wellness, Susan's comprehensive guide offers valuable information backed by research, allowing readers to effectively integrate red light into their daily routine.

"Microdosing: Macrobenefits in health and well-being. Your body in psychedelic and non-psychedelic substances."

In her most innovative work, Susan explores the fascinating world of microdosing and its impacts on health and wellness. This book provides a balanced and scientifically grounded view on the use of psychedelic and non-psychedelic substances in microdosing, offering a unique perspective on their potential benefit to mental and emotional health.

"High-Need Babies, The Untold Truth: The Ultimate Parenting Guide for High-Demanding Childs (English Edition)"

Susan McDowell embarks on the journey of parenting with her English-language play "High-Need Babies." This book provides a unique and comprehensive insight for parents facing the challenge of raising children with high demands. With empathy and wisdom, Susan guides parents through effective strategies and offers an enlightening perspective on the particular needs of these children.